Blueprint
for
Self-Care

**Creating Time, Space and a Peaceful
Healing Sanctuary for those in the
Helping Professions**

_____

Beverly Kyer

For speaking engagements:

email: kyergroupcorp@gmail.com

Phone: 925-709-3300

Travel Coordinator Email: mitchelljamal71@gmail.com

TABLE OF CONTENTS

INTRODUCTION   1

Step 1: Prepare   4

Step 2: Impact Control   13

Step 3: Bounce Back   18

Step 4: Say NO   22

Step 5: Evaluate   31

Step 6: Recharge   36

Step 7: Appreciate   42

Author's Corner   51

INTRODUCTION

Providing services and caregiving to struggling,

victimized and traumatized children, youth, adults and the

elderly is mentally and emotionally taxing. It can and will

wear our bodies out. The following is a seven point

Blueprint I developed to help promote Self-Care for your

health and wellness. Compassion Fatigue is a natural

outcome of the intense nature of the help we provide. We

each may feel the impact of secondary and vicarious

traumatic stress and burnout. However, we can take steps

to recover and increase our resilience for the ongoing

highly intense moments in our work. We can do this by

diligently taking preventative, release, recovery and restorative measures.

Many times I will hear from service providers that time, money and private space are in short supply given their particular circumstances. These are most often stated impediments to self-care. I have listed a few suggestions from myself and others from various fields of helping professionals who create opportunities for themselves. **Make these seven steps a consistent part of your life.**

P.I.B.S.E.R.A.

1. **Prepare** – Begin with a good night's sleep then start each day: Meditate/ Be intentional /Awareness of mind, body and spirit connection

2. **Impact control** – Ask yourself, Where am I in this moment? Mobilize strategies / breathe / have dual awareness; reduce toxic input.

3. **Bounce back** - Process and integrate/narrative/ Journal/breathe

4. **Say NO - STOP everything and take time for yourself**

5. **Evaluate -** Body scan (CHECK FOR PHYSICAL AND EMOTIONAL INJURIES) / breathe.

6. **Recharge -** Laughter / fun / prayer of thanksgiving / affection receive it and give it.

7. **Appreciate** - Artistic activity / view beauty / meditate on something wonderful/endorphins

<u>Step 1: Prepare</u>

PREPARE yourself each day with a brief period of

MEDITATION 5 – 10 MINUTES WILL DO (20 minutes

will come with practice).

Here are some practical tips you can implement today:

- Get a good restorative night's sleep.

- Settle down and quiet your mind at least one hour before bedtime and still your body with 3 or more slow deep breaths.

- Shut off the TV – especially the toxic news reports and programs.

- Choose a single sentence scripture or affirmation to repeat over and over verbally or mentally.

- Play non-lyrical music – this helps your mind to minimize internal dialogues and maximize the power of silence.

- Make a written list of all unfinished business. A to do list. By taking these concerns and putting them on paper, your mind enters a clear and calm, restful and regenerative state known as REM sleep.

- Enjoy some aroma therapy by rubbing a few drops of essential oils in the palm of your hand, then placing your hands over your nose, while breathing deeply as you lay down to sleep.

Each morning, **SET AN INTENTION FOR THE DAY** to accomplish 2-3 top priorities. YOUR HEALTH MAINTENANCE must always be one of your intentions. Make a written note of all tasks to be accomplished and be sure to check off what is completed. The brain loves to see check marks. Remind yourself daily of the connectedness of the mind, body, and spirit and that you must *GIVE ATTENTION TO THE TRIUNE YOU*

<u>Suggestions for step 1</u>

Use an area of your back yard (or sit near an open window) that is fragrant with flowers and pleasant to the eye. Early morning when the air is still relatively clear of automobile emissions is a good time to take some cleansing breaths and just sit quietly with a positive quote or an affirmation or a scripture to meditate on. Keep your thoughts completely in the present.

- When time is limited in the morning, dress for work then drive by your neighborhood park and take a short walk while meditating. Change from walking shoes to your work shoes when you return to your car. Do not walk fast enough to exert yourself and perspire. You simply wish to get some healthy blood circulation, cleansing breaths and to calm your nervous system.

- Sit quietly in a peaceful area of your apartment or on the front or back porch/balcony during a quiet time of the day or evening. Notice and enjoy the breeze in the trees and the chirping of birds.

- Sit up in bed first thing in the morning and declare this your time. Have your bible, prayer book or affirmation book and a note pad and pen on the bed stand. Also have a CD with a spiritual message or soothing music ready to just push the button and quietly reflect on the message. Begin your day with thanksgivings for the things you are happy about and grateful for. Read one of your chosen passages and or listen to a brief recording. Close your eyes and take some deep breaths and think on these messages. Embrace them. Soak them in. After about ten or more minutes, some ideas for the day will float into your mind. This experience is somewhat like receiving a download. You will know these are things you wish to do so write them down. When I do this exercise (from the comfort of a reclining reading chair I have in my bedroom), these down loads usually become my intentions for the day. The amazing thing about this practice is that it helps me stay on track of the really important things. This practice also works as a good reminder of things that have slipped my mind. This practice improves my memory which is very beneficial for those of you who like me are always multitasking.

- I personally like first thing in the morning when all else is quiet. I highly recommend to those of you who are morning people to rise before everyone else in the house and spend these moments calming yourself, mentally or verbally expressing gratitude, receiving your source and making intentions for your day under divine guidance.

- No matter your tasks facing you each day, work not to anticipate the worst case scenarios. Repeat to yourself, I will do my best AND I will be fine today. It is important to stay in the present and not focus on the events of future days. To do so is to overwhelm your own self. Follow the same thought processes for each of the suggestions for meditation.

- Take a few minutes and write in the lines provided your plan for creating a sanctuary space for your meditation time. Be thoughtful about what you want that will create a soothing and healing environment and bring some peace and joy to your day, each day.

- NOTES_____

_____

_____

_____

_____

_____

_____

_____

_____

_____

_____

_____

_____

Step 2: Impact Control

Prior to, during and post even the seemly least stressful situations, it is a good practice to always ask yourself **"WHERE AM I IN THIS MOMENT?"** This is a way of staying self-aware and taking care of yourself concurrent with the care you are giving to others. Traumatic stress *will* occur, however you now are in **CONTROL TO MANAGE AND MINIMIZE THE IMPACT** on yourself. Utilize the most convenient **STRESS MANAGEMENT TECHNIQUES** given time and space (e.g. you can do something tactical in the moment.) You may need to wait a while to have an opportunity to talk it out; however, embrace the process

ASAP.

Suggestions for step 2.

- I thought it a good idea to suggest limiting the amount of toxic and repetitive news reporting you allow to infiltrate your ears, your thoughts, your emotions and mood… I suggest the more bulleted forms of internet news, where you are able to select to view your choices of relevant information, and updates, without the bombardment of sensationalized tragedies, and/or anger provoking spins on current events.

- Take a moment before any interaction such as a client/patient contact, a site visit or a phone communication and check in with yourself. Even when the phone rings in your office and the ID window shows you the name of a particularly

challenging personality on the other line, take a
moment to prepare yourself. Ask yourself "where am
I in the moment?" "Am I okay?" "Am I ready for
this?" Take some breaths along with your self-
inventory.

- Take a moment to depersonalize the behavior you
  may anticipate experiencing from them. Remember
  the MOC perspective that their grief, fear and stress
  that drives their possibly undesirable behaviors, is not
  really about you. It is not personal. Granted their
  intent may be to make it a personal attack against
  you. However, you get to decide not to accept this
  invitation. Remember to check your personal
  boundaries here too. Respectfully and with kindness
  decide how people get to treat you. Next speak to

yourself: "I'm ok" "I accept myself" "I'm good";

"I've got this".

<u>Step 3: Bounce Back</u>

Two things need to happen to begin the inner work of recovery and healing. We need to process; or talk it out; release it with peers and in supervision. We also need to integrate which is being aware of the internal (physical) impact of the external (stressor) situation that is happening/has happened. Using the tools of "Narrative", "Body scanning" and "Journaling" can be quite helpful to process the triggering event.

Do not allow the negative content to fester inside of you. Do not repress the negative content and allow it to remain buried or stored inside of you while you pile on more and more distressing material over the course of the day(s).

Do a self-check or self-inventory along with proper breathing and the tense to relax exercise directed at the area(s) of your body where you are experiencing discomfort. This is helpful with integrating once you have made the connection between the external stressor and the internal (physical) impact that is happening to you.

Suggestions for step 3:

- Become knowledgeable about and aware of what is going on for you.

- Attend to your internal distresses using positive self-talk and deep slow breaths immediately and then get back to theirs.

- Remember the chaos is theirs not yours.

- Remember the pain is theirs not yours.

- Remember to take responsibility for the delivery of quality service, not the outcome.

- Remember to use reasonable expectations and fairness to how you measure on the job success.

- Remember to appreciate small successes.

- Remember **you** are as important as the service you are

giving.

• Breathe while remembering and visualizing a beautiful place or scene.

• Breathe while remembering an act of kindness done towards you.

• Breathe while thinking of someone you currently and actively love.

Step 4: Say NO

Learn to SAY NO! Which means STOP everything and take time out for you. Practice calendaring in some down periods for yourself at different junctures throughout the day AND some time off during the weekend. This is in addition to the time you give yourself to DECOMPRESS after a crisis. Make it a habit to be tenacious in guarding your time. People who you think will be disappointed or resentful because you said NO will get over it if they sincerely care about you and your wellbeing.

Suggestions for step 4

Saying no is the hardest thing to say for many of us. For some of us it is the way we are wired as helpers to over extend ourselves when we should stop and rest. We will actually allow someone to fill a ten or fifteen minutes we have to decompress to do something that can wait. Most concerning is that we do not take one day off or at least most of one day off during the week.

For many of us it is our cultural orientations. We have grown up with strong messages to always serve the needs of others before ourselves. I observed my parents working hard on jobs, at church, in the community and if a neighbor was struggling, they would be helping hands.

Later in life as an adult I would fill the weekend with household chores plus various obligatory activities that sent me back to work Monday mornings quite tired.

My suggestion for those with children at home is to consider grocery shopping one evening during the week when the super market is less crowed. I have always thought shopping on Saturdays was a nightmare and a terrible waste of a good day.

Try doing a load of laundry each morning. This way you don't have to use half of a precious day off doing laundry. I put a load in while getting ready for work. I threw the clothes in the dryer on the way out the door. I made folding the clothes one of my three children's after school chores. If you do not have a washer and dryer at home, (I did not have in home laundry at one point) use the same practice as shopping during the week. My children and I would do and check their homework in the Laundromat. To avoid over taxing myself on these nights I would either make sandwiches and soup or bring in Chinese food when my budget permitted. My goal again here was to have Saturdays free for fun and relaxation.

On your chosen weekend day off choose activities where your children can play themselves tired and you can sit observe and relax from time to time. Include a recreational activity for yourself also. The most important point here is to avoid allowing other people to fill up your time off unless they were there to join in the fun or relaxation. You may need to reevaluate your activities and decide what could be cut to make time for your best interest. Be very tenacious about protecting your time off.

Take a personal inventory here:

List three reasons why you find it difficult to say no

_____

_____

_____

_____

_____

_____

_____

_____

_____

_____

_____

Are these reasons golden cows? In other words, would saying no result in loss of life, home or health.

Yes._____   No._____   Why?

_____

_____

_____

_____

_____

_____

_____

_____

_____

_____

_____

What would it take for you to disaffirm the messages that prevent you from saying no when you need to take time out for yourself to rest and recharge?

_____

_____

_____

_____

_____

_____

_____

_____

_____

_____

_____

Some more points to consider about this matter of saying NO:

- People who really care about you will get over you saying "no".

- Consider that you will be a better person when you are feeling better

- Know that you will increase your on the job effectiveness, job satisfaction and quality of life when you consistently practice self-care.

For those operating life in the cultural messages given to us as young people, know that life when we were younger; life for our parents and grandparents had its difficulties. However life then was much less complex in terms of technologies that give people much greater access to us. In the Helping Professional systems, demands on the worker are ever increasing. We are living in a time when traumatic stressors relative to our service populations are more pervasive. There are many more critical demands that tax our energies and ware our bodies out. This calls on all service providers and caregivers to make self-care a top priority.

Step 5: Evaluate

Some of us are aware of a tensing in our bodies during stressful events. This restricts blood flow, causes some physical sensation, such as abdominal discomfort, which makes it difficult to focus. A beneficial skill is to use *A TENSE TO RELAX PROCESS.*

Where there is noticeable sensation in your body such as tightness, aches and pains, place your hand over the distressed area. Take two slow and deep breaths while focusing your breathing into that area. On the third inhalation tighten your right arm from the shoulder to your hand and hold tightly for two to three seconds. As you

exhaled relax fully and let your arm drop. Repeat these

four steps with your left arm, and then your right and left

leg from the balls of your feet, all the way up to your

thighs. Next do the trunk of your body. In seconds you

will *RELAX YOUR BODY AND CLEAR YOUR MIND.*

This method was based on research by Dr. Edmond

Jacobson:

SCAN YOUR BODY from head to foot for tightness

or aches. Notice any discomforting sensation after a

stressor. This is practicing BODY AWARENESS of where

stress attacks your body. Where ever you experience a

sensation and any emotion attached to that particular

sensation, place your hand over the area, focus your

thoughts on it and breathe into that area. Do this from

head to foot. This method helps you clear your body and mind of toxic blocks or build up.

Recognizing that breath is the window to the nervous system, I suggest you do two (2) minutes of DEEP AND SLOW BREATHING; inhaling to the count of three (3) and exhaling completely to the count of six (6). This method will relax your muscle tensions, regulate your heart rate and respiration, lower your blood pressure, help you manage your emotions and create inner peace both mentally and physically.

Suggestions for step 5:

Breath is something we take for granted. The air to breathe is always there so we do not think about it. Because we do not think much about it, we are usually unconscious of how shallow we breathe routinely. Here is where we necd many reminders to breathe using a slow, deep and rhythmic pattern of breathing to un-constrict our bodies, regulate our heart rate and calm our nervous system.

• Have your work place accountability partners cue you to breathe frequently throughout the day.

• Ask coworkers to cue you to breathe when they witness you in a crisis, even before or after a seemingly routine but difficult work situation.

• Put web alerts to pop up at intervals throughout the

work day and at home that cue you to take some deep and slow breaths.

• After experiencing a verbal or physical altercation or threat between/with clients; patients; inmates; you and your team of staff who were in that area where the disturbance happened, you should quickly gather and spend five (5) minutes doing a "tense-to-relax" exercise together. By doing this as a team, it encourages each member of the work team to take the impact of the experience serious and do some immediate self-care. In many ways it is the team supportively holding each member accountable for self-care.

• Following the same team work principal described for the tense to relax technique; the work team can alternately spend 5- 10 minutes doing body scanning.

<u>Step 6: Recharge</u>

It is highly beneficial to RECHARGE your energies after challenging times with activities that are filled with HUMOR AND FUN. Also speak to yourself (and your Creator) words of thanksgiving. Instead of repeating the negative things that happen, give thanks for what did not happen in the same situation. Shift your internal dialog to positives.

Giving affection and receiving it is also powerful in recharging the spirit and mind. The skin is the heaviest organ on the body. All sensory pathways lead to the surface of the skin. Hugging is magnificently calming. These activities change brain chemistry in a very positive way. They are like installing a fresh battery in a clock that is not able to move clock wise.

Suggestions for step 6:

Reconnect to, or build on and enhance, or develop a spiritual walk for your life. Remind yourself throughout your day that you are wonderfully created. You are doing the work the Creator chose you for. You are never alone. You are fully equipped. You are protected. You are deeply loved and appreciated by your creator for what you give to those you serve.

- Practice saying thank you for the small victories and thank you when situations and outcomes are less than desirable. Find the good in every situation. This may take a lot of practice. This may often require the input of shared insight from a co-worker(s) to see it, but the good is there.

- Join classes for meditation, yoga, qi-gong, and tai-chi--even rent videos to use at home.

- Have a SPA day including body massage; pedicure; manicure; facial. Beauty schools are inexpensive.

- See funny and uplifting movies as fast as they hit the screen.

- Attend music concerts. If for instance some notable entertainers is not in the budget, attend concerts and plays given at community theaters, programs and churches.

- Get a subscription to Netflix.com, Hulu.com or some great video streaming and watch family entertainment, spiritually based films, comedies, Stand-up Comedians and movies that leave you smiling.

- Gather often with friends that love to dance, love fun table games and activities and who make you laugh.

- Give affection to close loved ones and learn to receive it back to you.

This is not an exhaustive list. Drawing from this list and ideas of your own, what would be a plan just for you?:

_____

_____

_____

_____

_____

_____

_____

_____

_____

_____

_____

_____

_____

Step 7: Appreciate

A symptom of compassion fatigue is loss of libido; a loss of excitement and zeal for life. You may have lost interest in doing the things that gave you pleasure. Reignite these passions by *appreciating* beauty again. Don't wait until you feel like it; do it until you feel like it.

Be artistic even if you think you have limited talent. Visit or use media to gaze on panoramic scenery such as waterfalls, mountains, skies and seascapes. Indulge in music that delights your spirit. CREATE beautiful artistic works with paints, clay, needles, etc. The creative thinking and the activities of artist creation is a healing balm for

your spirit, mind and body.

Suggestions for step 7:

- Visit a botanicals garden and sculpture gardens frequently.

- Visit art studios.

- Visit the shore and enjoy the movement of the water.

- Hike in beautiful mountainous areas and our trail parks.

- Watch the sun rise in the mornings and/or set in the evenings.

- Indulge in classical music, gospel, jazz, rhythm and blues, Luther Vandross, Barry White...

- Use aroma therapy on your body with essential oils; in your house, with fragrant candle warmers.

- Soak in scented foaming baths with candle light and music.

- Make jewelry, pottery, various crafts (sign up for free introductory classes for crafts).

- Do photography.

- Garden and don't follow suit with your neighbors, create your own outdoors paradise.

- Paint on canvas; paint on plain white dishes; paint on fabric.

- Crochet; knit; sew; make something simple but colorful and beautiful.

- Write poetry or short stories.

- Rearrange a room; paint it; hang a beautiful mural of a scene that enchants you.

TAKE A MOMENT AND MAKE A LIST OF YOUR CHOICES FROM THIS LIST.

_____

_____

_____

_____

_____

_____

_____

_____

_____

_____

_____

_____

_____

Make a plan and share it with an accountability partner(s) make these intentions and make them healthy habits for self-care.

_____

_____

_____

_____

_____

_____

_____

_____

_____

_____

_____

Pertinent Notes To Live By:

_____

_____

_____

_____

_____

_____

_____

_____

_____

_____

_____

_____

_____

_____

_____

Author's Corner

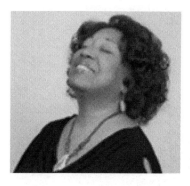

Beverly Kyer is highly sought after speaker, trainer and coach on Compassion Fatigue. She has a Master's Degree in Social Work and is in the Academy of Certified Social Workers. She has postgraduate certificates and three plus decades of experience in integrated Approach to Readjustment Counseling; Post Traumatic Stress Disorder; Social Research for the mentally ill and Employee Assistance Program Coordination.

Beverly became a Clinical Social Worker for Pediatric Oncology; Vietnam Veterans; Psychiatry and Child Welfare. She spent a major portion of her career with the Veterans Administration Veteran's Outreach Center and Medical Center in Bronx New York. Beverly also spent more than a decade in Foster Care, and five years as an urban High School Counselor providing emotional and psychological support for students and staff.

Two episodes of Heart Failure lead Beverly to make a major downshift in her life by resigning from full time employment; joining the self-employed and devoting her efforts to help others who work in highly stressful environments. Beverly Lectures around the country on Compassion Fatigue AKA Secondary and Vicarious Traumatic Stress.

Beverly has two natural sons and an adopted daughter;

each of whom are independent adults, and really considerate and compassionate people. Beverly makes her home in Northern California in a quiet cul-de-sac near the Delta. Oil painting, music, movies and good books are among her passions.

For speaking engagements:

email: kyergroupcorp@gmail.com

Phone: 925-709-3300

Travel Coordinator Email: mitchelljamal71@gmail.com

Made in the USA
Columbia, SC
08 February 2020